Overweight and Weightloss Facts Report

by Martha Johnson

Overweight and Weight loss is challenging to many people. Being over weight often contributes to disease. Do you really know that you are over weight or do you know how much overweight you are? The Center for Disease and Prevention gives helpful insight on how you may lose weight to live a healthy lifestyle.
Set realistic goals for yourself and get started living a healthier lifestyle.

Table of Contents

1. Are you Overweight?

How do I know if I'm overweight or obese?

Body Mass Index

You can find out your BMI by using this chart.
Find out your body mass index (BMI). BMI is a measure of body fat based on height and weight.
People with a BMI of 25 to 29.9 are considered overweight. People with a BMI of 30 or more are considered obese.

To use the table, find the appropriate height in the left-hand column labeled Height. Move across to a given weight (in pounds). The number at the top of the column is the BMI at that height and weight.
Pounds have been rounded off.

BMI	19	20	21	22	23	24	25	26	27	28	29	30	31	32	33	34	35
Height (inches)							Body Weight (pounds)										
58	91	96	100	105	110	115	119	124	129	134	138	143	148	153	158	162	167
59	94	99	104	109	114	119	124	128	133	138	143	148	153	158	163	168	173
60	97	102	107	112	118	123	128	133	138	143	148	153	158	163	168	174	179
61	100	106	111	116	122	127	132	137	143	148	153	158	164	169	174	180	185
62	104	109	115	120	126	131	136	142	147	153	158	164	169	175	180	186	191
63	107	113	118	124	130	135	141	146	152	158	163	169	175	180	186	191	197
64	110	116	122	128	134	140	145	151	157	163	169	174	180	186	192	197	204
65	114	120	126	132	138	144	150	156	162	168	174	180	186	192	198	204	210
66	118	124	130	136	142	148	155	161	167	173	179	186	192	198	204	210	216
67	121	127	134	140	146	153	159	166	172	178	185	191	198	204	211	217	223
68	125	131	138	144	151	158	164	171	177	184	190	197	203	210	216	223	230
69	128	135	142	149	155	162	169	176	182	189	196	203	209	216	223	230	236
70	132	139	146	153	160	167	174	181	188	195	202	209	216	222	229	236	243
71	136	143	150	157	165	172	179	186	193	200	208	215	222	229	236	243	250
72	140	147	154	162	169	177	184	191	199	206	213	221	228	235	242	250	258
73	144	151	159	166	174	182	189	197	204	212	219	227	235	242	250	257	265
74	148	155	163	171	179	186	194	202	210	218	225	233	241	249	256	264	272
75	152	160	168	176	184	192	200	208	216	224	232	240	248	256	264	272	279
76	156	164	172	180	189	197	205	213	221	230	238	246	254	263	271	279	287

BMI	36	37	38	39	40	41	42	43	44	45	46	47	48	49	50	51	52	53	54
Height (inches)	Body Weight (pounds)																		
58	172	177	181	186	191	196	201	205	210	215	220	224	229	234	239	244	248	253	258
59	178	183	188	193	198	203	208	212	217	222	227	232	237	242	247	252	257	262	267
60	184	189	194	199	204	209	215	220	225	230	235	240	245	250	255	261	266	271	276
61	190	195	201	206	211	217	222	227	232	238	243	248	254	259	264	269	275	280	285
62	196	202	207	213	218	224	229	235	240	246	251	256	262	267	273	278	284	289	295
63	203	208	214	220	225	231	237	242	248	254	259	265	270	278	282	287	293	299	304
64	209	215	221	227	232	238	244	250	256	262	267	273	279	285	291	296	302	308	314
65	216	222	228	234	240	246	252	258	264	270	276	282	288	294	300	306	312	318	324
66	223	229	235	241	247	253	260	266	272	278	284	291	297	303	309	315	322	328	334
67	230	236	242	249	255	261	268	274	280	287	293	299	306	312	319	325	331	338	344
68	236	243	249	256	262	269	276	282	289	295	302	308	315	322	328	335	341	348	354
69	243	250	257	263	270	277	284	291	297	304	311	318	324	331	338	345	351	358	365
70	250	257	264	271	278	285	292	299	306	313	320	327	334	341	348	355	362	369	376
71	257	265	272	279	286	293	301	308	315	322	329	338	343	351	358	365	372	379	386
72	265	272	279	287	294	302	309	316	324	331	338	346	353	361	368	375	383	390	397
73	272	280	288	295	302	310	318	325	333	340	348	355	363	371	378	386	393	401	408
74	280	287	295	303	311	319	326	334	342	350	358	365	373	381	389	396	404	412	420
75	287	295	303	311	319	327	335	343	351	359	367	375	383	391	399	407	415	423	431
76	295	304	312	320	328	336	344	353	361	369	377	385	394	402	410	418	426	435	443

Assessment of weight and health risk involves using three key measures:

1. Body mass index (BMI)
2. Waist circumference
3. Risk factors for diseases and conditions associated with obesity

Body Mass Index (BMI)

BMI is a useful measure of overweight and obesity. It is calculated from your height and weight. BMI is an estimate of body fat and a good gauge of your risk for diseases that can occur with more body fat. The higher your BMI, the higher your risk for certain diseases such as heart disease, high blood pressure, type 2 diabetes, gallstones, breathing problems, and certain cancers.

Although BMI can be used for most men and women, it does have some limits: It may overestimate body fat in athletes and others who have a muscular build.

It may underestimate body fat in older persons and others who have lost muscle.
Measuring waist circumference helps screen for possible health risks that come with overweight and obesity. If most of your fat is around your waist rather than at your hips, you're at a higher risk for heart disease and type 2 diabetes. This risk goes up with a waist size that is greater than 35 inches for women or greater than 40 inches for men. To correctly measure your waist, stand and place a tape measure around your middle, just above your hipbones. Measure your waist just after you breathe out.

1. What Causes Overweight and Obesity?

You can become overweight or obese when you eat more calories (KAL-oh-rees) than you use. A calorie is a unit of energy in the food you eat. Your body needs this energy to function and to be active. But if you take in more energy than your body uses, you will gain weight.

Many factors can play a role in becoming overweight or obese. These factors include:

- Behaviors, such as eating too many calories or not getting enough physical activity
- Environment and culture
- Genes

Overweight and obesity problems keep getting worse in the United States. Some cultural reasons for this include:

- Bigger portion sizes

- Little time to exercise or cook healthy meals

Using cars to get places instead of walking

Watch Your Weight

To stay at a healthy weight, balance the calories you eat with the calories you burn (use up). To lose weight, you need to use more calories than you eat. A healthy diet and physical activity can help you control your weight.

Calories are a measure of the energy in the foods you eat. You burn calories when you are physically active.
A 154-pound man (5' 10") will use up about the number of calories listed doing each activity below. **Those who weigh more will use more calories, and those who weigh less will use fewer.**

Moderate physical activities:	Approximate calories used by a 154 pound man In 1 hour	In 30 minutes
Hiking	370	185
Light gardening/yard work	330	165
Dancing	330	165
Golf (walking and carrying clubs)	330	165
Bicycling (less than 10 miles per hour)	290	145
Walking (3 ½ miles per hour)	280	140
Weight training (general light workout)	220	110
Stretching	180	90
Vigorous physical activities:	**In 1 hour**	**In 30 minutes**
Running/jogging (5 miles per hour)	590	295
Bicycling (more than 10 miles per hour)	590	295
Swimming (slow freestyle laps)	510	255
Aerobics	480	240
Walking (4 ½ miles per hour)	460	230
Heavy yard work (chopping wood)	440	220
Weight lifting (vigorous effort)	440	220
Basketball (vigorous)	440	220

What can losing weight do for me?

If you are overweight or obese, losing weight can lower your risk for serious health conditions like:

- Type 2 diabetes
- Heart disease
- High blood pressure
- Early death

Plus, eating healthy and being physically active can give you more energy throughout the day. Move more and eat healthy foods to help:

- Lower your blood pressure
- Lower your blood sugar
- Raise your "good" cholesterol
- Lower your "bad" cholesterol

You may start to see these benefits by losing just 5 to 10 percent of your body weight. For example, if you are 200 pounds, this could mean losing as little as 10 pounds.

Take Action!

Make a promise to eat well, move more, and get support from family and friends. If you need to lose weight, do it slowly over time.

Remember that to lose weight, you need to eat fewer calories than you burn.

2. Setting Realistic Goals

Set realistic goals.
Start out by setting small goals, like:

- I want to lose 1 to 2 pounds a week.
- I will add 10 minutes of physical activity to my daily routine.
- I will avoid second helpings of meals this week.

Keep a food and activity diary.
Write down:

- When you eat
- What you eat
- How much you eat
- Your physical activity

Keep a food and activity diary. When you know your habits, it's easier to make changes.

_Move more to balance the calories you take in with the calories you use.

- Aim for 2 hours and 30 minutes of activity a week.
- Try to be active for 30 minutes 5 times a week.
- If you don't have time for 30 minutes of activity, get moving for shorter 10-minute periods throughout the day.

Remember that some physical activity is better than none. Check out these resources for tips and ideas:

Active at Any Size.WOULD you like to be more physically active, but are not sure if you can do it?

Good news-if you are a very large person, **you _can_ be physically active**-and you can have fun and feel good doing it.

THERE may be special challenges for very large people who are physically active. You may not be able to bend or move in the same way that other people can. It may be hard to find clothes and equipment for exercising. You may feel self-conscious being physically active around other people.

Facing these challenges is hard-but it can be done! The information in this booklet may help you start being more active and healthier-**no matter what your size!**

What Kind of Activity Should I do?

To get the health benefits of physical activity, do a combination of aerobic and muscle-strengthening activities.

9

- **Aerobic** ("air-OH-bik") activities make you breathe harder and cause your heart to beat faster. Walking fast is an example of aerobic activity.

Muscle-strengthening activities make your muscles stronger. Muscle-strengthening activities include lifting weights and using exercise bands.

Eat Healthy

Here are some easy ways you can eat healthy.

- Choose fat-free or low-fat versions of your favorite foods.
- Drink water or fat-free milk instead of soda or other sugary drinks.
- Fill half your plate with vegetables and fruit.
- When you eat out, ask for sauces or dressings "on the side" so you can control how much you use.

Eat smaller portions.

Eating healthy food is important. But you also need to pay attention to **how much** food you eat.

- Start the day with a healthy breakfast.
- Eat small, healthy snacks during the day. This will keep you from overeating at mealtimes.
- Put a small amount of food in a bowl instead of eating out of the package or container.
- Serve food on plates and leave the main dish on the stove. You will be less tempted to go back for seconds.
- If you are eating out, only eat half of your meal. Take the other half home.
- Read the label to find out how many servings are in a package. There may be more than one!
- Eat slowly – this will give you time to feel full.
- Don't eat in front of the TV. It's harder to keep track of how much you are eating.

Ask your doctor for help.
You may also want to talk to a doctor or nurse about different ways to lose weight. Your doctor can explain your options, like joining a weight-loss program.

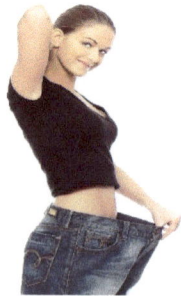

People who want to lose a large amount of weight (more than 5 percent of their body weight)—and people who want to keep off the weight that they've lost may need to be physically active for more than 300 minutes of moderate-intensity activity each week.

Key Recommendations (From the *Clinical Guidelines on the Identification, Evaluation and Treatment of Overweight and Obesity in Adults: Evidence Report*, 1998)

- Weight loss to lower elevated blood pressure in overweight and obese persons with high blood pressure.
- Weight loss to lower elevated levels of total cholesterol, LDL-cholesterol, and triglycerides, and to raise low levels of HDL-cholesterol, in overweight and obese persons with dyslipidemia.
- Weight loss to lower elevated blood glucose levels in overweight and obese persons with type 2 diabetes.
- Use the BMI to assess overweight and obesity. Body weight alone can be used to follow weight loss and to determine the effectiveness of therapy.
- Use the BMI to classify overweight and obesity and to estimate relative risk of disease compared to normal weight.
- The waist circumference should be used to assess abdominal fat content.
- The initial goal of weight-loss therapy should be to reduce body weight by about 10 percent from baseline. With success, and if warranted, further weight loss can be attempted.
- Weight loss should be about 1 to 2 pounds per week for a period of 6 months, with the subsequent strategy based on the amount of weight lost.
- Low-calorie diets (LCD) for weight loss in overweight and obese persons. Reducing fat as part of an LCD is a practical way to reduce calories.
- Reducing dietary fat alone without reducing calories is not sufficient for weight loss. However, reducing dietary fat, along with reducing dietary carbohydrates, can help reduce calories.
- A diet that is individually planned to help create a deficit of 500 to 1,000 kcal/day should be an intregal part of any program aimed at achieving a weight loss of 1 to 2 pounds per week.
- Physical activity should be part of a comprehensive weight loss therapy and weight control program because it (1) modestly contributes to weight loss in overweight and obese adults, (2) may decrease abdominal fat, (3) increases cardio respiratory fitness, and (4) may help with maintenance of weight loss.
- Physical activity should be an integral part of weight-loss therapy and weight maintenance. Initially, moderate levels of physical activity for 30 to 45 minutes, 3 to 5 days a week, should be encouraged. All adults should set a long-term goal to accumulate at least 30 minutes or more of moderate-intensity physical activity on most, and preferably all, days of the week.
- The combination of a reduced-calorie diet and increased physical activity is recommended, because it produces weight loss that also may result in decreases in abdominal fat and increases in cardio respiratory fitness.
- Behavior therapy is a useful adjunct when incorporated into treatment for weight loss and weight maintenance.
- Weight-loss and weight-maintenance therapy should employ the combination of LCDs, increased physical activity, and behavior therapy.

- After successful weight loss, the likelihood of weight-loss maintenance is enhanced by a program consisting of dietary therapy, physical activity, and behavior therapy, which should be continued indefinitely. Drug therapy also can be used. However, drug safety and efficacy beyond 1 year of total treatment have not been established.
- A weight maintenance program should be a priority after the initial 6 months of weight-loss therapy.

Do You know Some of Health Risks of Obesity?

What is type 2 diabetes?

Type 2 diabetes is a disease in which blood sugar levels are above normal. High blood sugar is a major cause of heart disease, kidney disease, stroke, amputation, and blindness. In 2009, diabetes was the seventh leading cause of death in the United States.

Type 2 diabetes is the most common type of diabetes. Family history and genes play a large role in type 2 diabetes. Other risk factors include a low activity level, poor diet, and excess body weight around the waist. In the United States, type 2 diabetes is more common among blacks, Latinos, and American Indians than among whites.

How is type 2 diabetes linked to overweight?

About 80 percent of people with type 2 diabetes are overweight or obese. It isn't clear why people who are overweight are more likely to develop this disease. It may be that being overweight causes cells to change, making them resistant to the hormone insulin. Insulin carries sugar from blood to the cells, where it is used for energy. When a person is insulin resistant, blood sugar cannot be taken up by the cells, resulting in high blood sugar. In addition, the cells that produce insulin must work extra hard to try to keep blood sugar normal. This may cause these cells to gradually fail.

How can weight loss help?

If you are at risk for type 2 diabetes, losing weight may help prevent or delay the onset of diabetes. If you have type 2 diabetes, losing weight and becoming more physically active can help you control your blood sugar levels and prevent or delay health problems. Losing weight and exercising more may also allow you to reduce the a
mount of diabetes medicine you take.

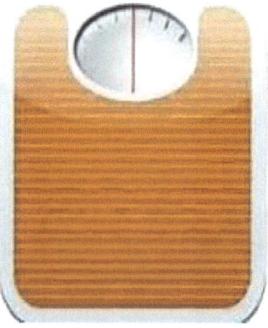

What is heart disease?

Heart disease is a term used to describe several problems that may affect your heart. The most common type of problem happens when a blood vessel that carries blood to the heart becomes hard and narrow. This may keep the heart from getting all the blood it needs. Other problems may affect how well the heart pumps. If you have heart disease, you may suffer from a heart attack, heart failure, sudden cardiac death, angina (chest pain), or abnormal heart rhythm. Heart disease is the leading cause of death in the United States.

How is heart disease linked to overweight?

People who are overweight or obese often have health problems that may increase the risk for heart disease. These health problems include high blood pressure, high cholesterol, and high blood sugar. In addition, excess weight may cause changes to your heart that make it work harder to send blood to all the cells in your body.

How can weight loss help?

Losing 5 to 10 percent of your weight may lower your chances of developing heart disease. If you weigh 200 pounds, this means losing as little as 10 pounds. Weight loss may improve blood pressure, cholesterol levels, and blood flow.

Measure	Target
Target BMI	18.5–24.9
Waist size	Men: less than 40 in. Women: less than 35 in.
Blood pressure	120/80 mm Hg or less
LDL (bad cholesterol)	Less than 100 mg/dL
HDL (good cholesterol)	Men: more than 40 mg/dL Women: more than 50 mg/dL
Triglycerides	Less than 150 mg/dL
Blood sugar (fasting)	Less than 100 mg/dL

Stroke

What is a stroke?

A stroke happens when the flow of blood to a part of your brain stops, causing brain cells to die. The most common type of stroke, called ischemic stroke, occurs when a blood clot blocks an artery that carries blood to the brain. Another type of stroke, called hemorrhagic stroke, happens when a blood vessel in the brain bursts.

How are strokes linked to overweight?

Overweight and obesity are known to increase blood pressure. High blood pressure is the leading cause of strokes. Excess weight also increases your chances of developing other problems linked to strokes, including high cholesterol, high blood sugar, and heart disease.

How can weight loss help?

One of the most important things you can do to reduce your stroke risk is to keep your blood pressure under control. Losing weight may help you lower your blood pressure. It may also improve your cholesterol and blood sugar, which may then lower your risk for stroke.

What kinds of cancers are linked to overweight and obesity?

Being overweight increases the risk of developing certain cancers, including the following :

- breast, after menopause
- colon and rectum
- endometrium (lining of the uterus)
- gallbladder
- kidney

What is cancer?

Cancer occurs when cells in one part of the body, such as the colon, grow abnormally or out of control. The cancerous cells sometimes spread to other parts of the body, such as the liver. Cancer is the second leading cause of death in the United States.

How is cancer linked to overweight?

Gaining weight as an adult increases the risk for several cancers, even if the weight gain doesn't result in overweight or obesity. It isn't known exactly how being overweight increases cancer risk. Fat cells may release hormones that affect cell growth, leading to cancer. Also, eating or physical activity habits that may lead to being overweight may also contribute to cancer risk.

How can weight loss help?

Avoiding weight gain may prevent a rise in cancer risk. Healthy eating and physical activity habits may lower cancer risk. Weight loss may also lower your risk, although studies have been inconclusive.

What is sleep apnea?

Sleep apnea is a condition in which a person has one or more pauses in breathing during sleep. A person who has sleep apnea may suffer from daytime sleepiness, difficulty focusing, and even heart failure.

How is sleep apnea linked to overweight?

Obesity is the most important risk factor for sleep apnea. A person who is overweight may have more fat stored around his or her neck. This may make the airway smaller. A smaller airway can make breathing difficult or loud (because of snoring), or breathing may stop altogether for short periods of time. In addition, fat stored in the neck and throughout the body may produce substances that cause inflammation. Inflammation in the neck is a risk factor for sleep apnea.

How can weight loss help?

Weight loss usually improves sleep apnea. Weight loss may help to decrease neck size and lessen inflammation.

What is osteoarthritis?

Osteoarthritis is a common health problem that causes pain and stiffness in your joints. Osteoarthritis is often related to aging or to an injury, and most often affects the joints of the hands, knees, hips, and lower back.

How is osteoarthritis linked to overweight?

Being overweight is one of the risk factors for osteoarthritis, along with joint injury, older age, and genetic factors. Extra weight may place extra pressure on joints and cartilage (the hard but slippery tissue that covers the ends of your bones at a joint), causing them to wear away. In addition, people with more body fat may have higher blood levels of substances that cause inflammation. Inflamed joints may raise the risk for osteoarthritis.

How can weight loss help?

For those who are overweight or obese, losing weight may help reduce the risk of developing osteoarthritis. Weight loss of at least 5 percent of your body weight may decrease stress on your knees, hips, and lower back and lessen inflammation in your body.

If you have osteoarthritis, losing weight may help improve your symptoms. Research also shows that exercise is one of the best treatments for osteoarthritis. Exercise can improve mood, decrease pain, and increase flexibility.

What is fatty liver disease?

Fatty liver disease, also known as nonalcoholic steatohepatitis (NASH), occurs when fat builds up in the liver and causes injury. Fatty liver disease may lead to severe liver damage, cirrhosis (scar tissue), or even liver failure.   15

Fatty liver disease usually produces mild or no symptoms. It is like alcoholic liver disease, but it isn't caused by alcohol and can occur in people who drink little or no alcohol.

How is fatty liver disease linked to overweight?

The cause of fatty liver disease is still not known. The disease most often affects people who are middle-aged, overweight or obese, and/or diabetic. Fatty liver disease may also affect children.

How can weight loss help?

Although there is no specific treatment for fatty liver disease, patients are generally advised to lose weight, eat a healthy diet, increase physical activity, and avoid drinking alcohol. If you have fatty liver disease, lowering your body weight to a healthy range may improve liver tests and reverse the disease to some extent.

What is kidney disease?

Your kidneys are two bean-shaped organs that filter blood, removing extra water and waste products, which become urine. Your kidneys also help control blood pressure so that your body can stay healthy.

Kidney disease means that the kidneys are damaged and can't filter blood like they should. This damage can cause wastes to build up in the body. It can also cause other problems that can harm your health.

How is kidney disease linked to overweight?

Obesity increases the risk of diabetes and high blood pressure, the most common causes of chronic kidney disease. Recent studies suggest that even in the absence of these risks, obesity itself may promote chronic kidney disease and quicken its progress.

How can weight loss help?

If you are in the early stages of chronic kidney disease, losing weight may slow the disease and keep your kidneys healthier longer. You should also choose foods with less salt (sodium), keep your blood pressure under control, and keep your blood glucose in the target range.

Overweight and obesity raise the risk of health problems for both mother and baby that may occur during pregnancy. Pregnant women who are overweight or obese may have an increased risk for

- developing gestational diabetes (high blood sugar during pregnancy)
- having preeclampsia (high blood pressure during pregnancy that can cause severe problems for both mother and baby if left untreated)
- needing a C-section and, as a result, taking longer to recover after giving birth

Babies of overweight or obese mothers are at an increased risk of being born too soon, being stillborn (dead in the womb after 20 weeks of pregnancy), and having neural tube defects (defects of the brain and spinal cord).

How many pounds should I gain during pregnancy?

Guidelines from the Institute of Medicine and the National Research Council, issued in 2009, recommend the following amount of weight gain during pregnancy

Pre-pregnancy Weight	Amount to Gain
Underweight (BMI < 18.5)	28–40 lbs.
Normal Weight (BMI 18.5–24.9)	25–35 lbs.
Overweight (BMI 25–29.9)	15–25 lbs.
Obesity (BMI 30+)	11–20 lbs.

How are pregnancy problems linked to overweight?

Pregnant women who are overweight are more likely to develop insulin resistance, high blood sugar, and high blood pressure. Overweight also increases the risks associated with surgery and anesthesia, and severe obesity increases surgery time and blood loss.

Gaining too much weight during pregnancy can have long-term effects for both mother and child. These effects include that the mother will have overweight or obesity after the child is born. Another risk is that the baby may gain too much weight later as a child or as an adult.

If you are pregnant, check the sidebar for general guidelines about weight gain. Talk to your health care provider about how much weight gain is right for you during pregnancy.

How can weight loss help?

If you are overweight or obese and would like to become pregnant, talk to your health care provider about losing weight first. Reaching a normal weight before becoming pregnant may reduce your chances of developing weight-related problems. Pregnant women who are overweight or obese should speak with their health care provider about limiting weight gain and being physically active during pregnancy.

Losing excess weight after delivery may help women reduce their health risks. For example, if a woman developed gestational diabetes, losing weight may lower her risk of developing diabetes later in life.

How can I lower my risk of having health problems related to overweight and obesity?

If you are considered to be overweight, losing as little as 5 percent of your body weight may lower your risk for several diseases, including heart disease and type 2 diabetes. If you weigh 200 pounds, this means losing 10 pounds. Slow and steady weight loss of 1/2 to 2 pounds per week, and not more than 3 pounds per week, is the safest way to lose weight.

Federal guidelines on physical activity recommend that you get at least 150 minutes a week of moderate aerobic activity (like biking or brisk walking). To lose weight, or to maintain weight loss, you may need to be active for up to 300 minutes per week. You also need to do activities to strengthen muscles (like push-ups or sit-ups) at least twice a week. See the Resources section for a hyper link to these guidelines.

Federal dietary guidelines and the MyPlate website recommend many tips for healthy eating that may also help you control your weight (see the Resources section for hyper links). Here are a few examples:

- Make half of your plate fruits and vegetables.
- Replace unrefined grains (white bread, pasta, white rice) with whole-grain options (whole wheat bread, brown rice, oatmeal).

Enjoy lean sources of protein, such as lean meats, seafood, beans and peas, soy, nuts, and seeds.

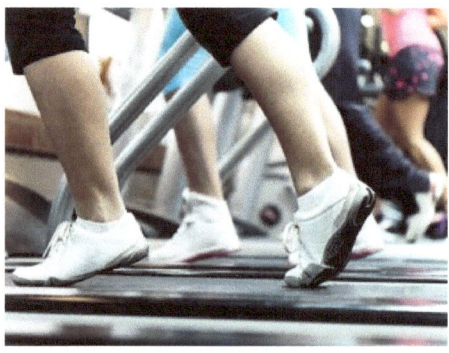

Resources:
Weight control Information Network
Center for Disease Prevention

The Benefits of Physical Activity

Regular physical activity is one of the most important things you can do for your health. It can help:

*Control your weight
*Reduce your risk of cardiovascular disease
*Reduce your risk for type 2 diabetes and metabolic syndrome
*Reduce your risk of some cancers
*Strengthen your bones and muscles
*Improve your mental health and mood
*Improve your ability to do daily activities and prevent falls,
  if you're an older adult
*Increase your chances of living longer

If you're not sure about becoming active or boosting your level of

physicalactivitybecause you're afraid of getting hurt, the good news is that **moderate intensity aerobic activity**, like brisk walking, is generally **safe for most people**.

Start slowly. Cardiac events, such as a heart attack, are rare during physical activity. But the risk does go up when you suddenly become much more active than usual. For example, you can put yourself at risk if you don't usually get much physical activity and then all of a sudden do vigorous-intensity aerobic activity, like shoveling snow. That's why it's important to start slowly and gradually increase your level of activity.

If you have a chronic health condition such as arthritis, diabetes, or heart disease, talk with your doctor to find out if your condition limits, in any way, your ability to be active. Then, work with your doctor to come up with a physical activity plan that matches your abilities. If your condition stops you from meeting the minimum *Guidelines*, try to do as much as you can. What's important is that you avoid being inactive. Even 60 minutes a week of moderate-intensity aerobic activity is good for you.

The bottom line is – the health benefits of physical activity far outweigh the risks of getting hurt.

Controlling Your Weight
Looking to get to or stay at a healthy weight? Both diet and physical activity play a critical role in controlling your weight. You gain weight when the calories you burn, including those burned during physical activity, are less than the calories you eat or drink. For more information see our section on balancing calories. When it comes to weight management, people vary greatly in how much physical activity they need. You may need to be more active than others to achieve or maintain a healthy weight.

To maintain your weight: Work your way up to 150 minutes of moderate-intensityaerobic activity, 75 minutes of vigorous-intensity aerobic activity, or an equivalentmix of the two each week. Strong scientific evidence shows that physical activity can help you maintain your weight over time. However, the exact amount of physical activity needed to do this is not clear since it varies greatly from person to person. It's possible that you may need to do more than the equivalent of 150 minutes of moderate-intensity activity a week to maintain your weight.

To lose weight and keep it off: You will need a high amount of physical activity unless you also adjust your diet and reduce the amount of calories you're eating and drinking. Getting to and staying at a healthy weight requires both regular physical activity and a healthy eating plan. The CDC has some great tools and information about nutrition, physical activity and weight loss.

Reduction in Your Risk of Cardiovascular Disease, Diabetes and Some Cancers

Reduce Your Risk of Cardiovascular Disease

Heart disease and stroke are two of the leading causes of death in the United States. But following the Guidelines and getting at least 150 minutes a week (2 hours and 30 minutes) of moderate-intensity aerobic activity can put you at a lower risk for these diseases. You can reduce your risk even further with more physical activity. Regular physical activity can also lower your blood pressure and improve your cholesterol levels.

Reduce your risk of Type 2 Diabetes and Metabolic Syndrome

Regular physical activity can reduce your risk of developing type 2 diabetes and metabolic syndrome. Metabolic syndrome is a condition in which you have some combination of too much fat around the waist, high blood pressure, low HDL cholesterol, high triglycerides, or high blood sugar. Research shows that lower rates of these conditions are seen with 120 to 150 minutes (2 hours to 2 hours and 30 minutes) a week of at least moderate-intensity aerobic activity. And the more physical activity you do, the lower your risk will be.

Already have type 2 diabetes? Regular physical activity can help control your blood glucose levels.

Reduce Your Risk of Some Cancers

Being physically active lowers your risk for two types of cancer: colon and breast. Research shows that:

- Physically active people have a lower risk of colon cancer than do people who are not active.
- Physically active women have a lower risk of breast cancer than do people who are not active.

Reduce your risk of endometrial and lung cancer. Although the research is not yet final, some findings suggest that your risk of endometrial cancer and lung cancer may be lower if you get regular physical activity compared to people who are not active.

Improve your quality of life. If you are a cancer survivor, research shows that getting regular physical activity not only helps give you a better quality of life, but also improves your physical fitness.

Strengthening Your Bones and Muscles

As you age, it's important to protect your bones, joints and muscles. Not only do theysupport yourbody and help you move, but keeping bones, joints and muscles healthy can help ensure that you're able to do your daily activities and be physically active. Research shows that doing **aerobic, muscle-strengthening and bone-strengthening physical activity** of at least a moderately-intense level **can slow the loss of bone density** that comes with age.

Hip fracture is a serious health condition that can have life-changing negative effects, especially if you're an older adult. But research shows that people who do 120 to 300 minutes of at least moderate-intensity aerobic activity each week have a lower risk of hip fracture.

Regular physical activity helps with arthritis and other conditions affecting the joints. If you have arthritis, research shows that doing 130 to 150 (2 hours and 10 minutes to 2 hours and 30 minutes) a week of moderate-intensity, low-impact aerobic activity can not only improve your ability to manage pain and do everyday tasks, but it can also make your quality of life better.

Build strong, healthy muscles. Muscle-strengthening activities can help you increase or maintainyour muscle mass and strength. Slowly increasing the amount of weight and number of repetitions you do will give you even more benefits, no matter your age.

Improve Your Mental Health and Mood

Regular physical activity can help keep your thinking, learning, and judgment skills sharp as you age. It can also reduce your risk of depression and may help you sleep better. Research has shown that doing aerobic or a mix of aerobic and muscle-strengthening activities 3 to 5 times a week for 30 to 60 minutes can give you these mental health benefits. Some scientific evidence has also shown that even lower levels of physical activity can be beneficial.

Improve Your Ability to do Daily Activities and Prevent Falls

A functional limitation is a loss of the ability to do everyday activities such as climbing stairs, grocery shopping, or playing with your grandchildren. **How does this relate to physical activity?** If you're a physically active middle-aged or older adult, you have a lower risk of functional limitations than people who are inactive

Already have trouble doing some of your everyday activities? Aerobic and muscle-strengthening activities can help improve your ability to do these types of tasks.

Are you an older adult who is at risk for falls? Research shows that doing **balance** and **muscle-strengthening activities** each week along with **moderate-intensity aerobic activity**, like brisk walking, can help reduce your risk of falling.

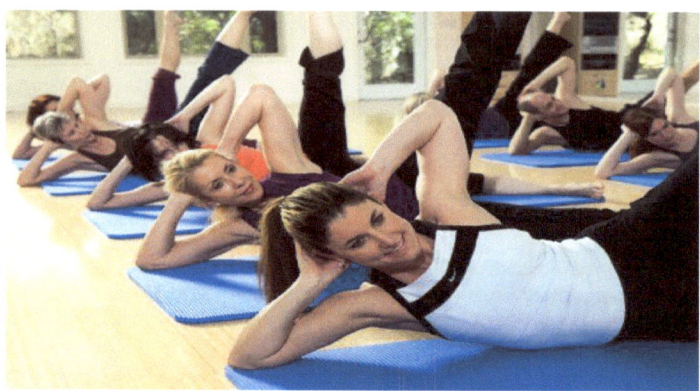

How Much Exercise Should I do for Losing weight and Does the Type Matter?

How much physical activity do I need to do to lose weight?

If you want to lose a substantial (more than 5 percent of body weight) amount of weight, you need a high amount of physical activity unless you also lower calorie intake. This is also the case if you are trying to keep the weight off. Many people need to do more than 300 minutes of moderate-intensity activity a week to meet weight-control goals.

Does the type of physical activity I choose matter?

Yes! Engaging in different types of physical activity is important to overall physical fitness. Your fitness routine should include aerobic and strength-training activities, and may also include stretching activities.

Aerobic activities

These activities move large muscles in your arms, legs, and hips over and over again. Examples include walking, jogging, bicycling, swimming, and tennis.

Strength-training activities

These activities increase the strength and endurance of your muscles. Examples of strength-training activities include working out with weight machines, free weights, and resistance bands. (A resistance band looks like a giant rubber band. You can buy one at a sporting goods store.) Push-ups and sit-ups are examples of strength-training activities you can do without any equipment. You also can use soup cans to work out your arms.

Aim to do strength-training activities at least twice a week. In each strength-training session, you should do 8 to 10 different activities using the different muscle groups throughout your body, such as the muscles in your abdomen, chest, arms, and legs. Repeat each activity 8 to 12 times, using a weight or resistance that will make you feel tired. When you do strength-training activities, slowly increase the amount of weight or resistance that you use. Also, allow one day in between sessions to avoid excess strain on your muscles and joints.

Stretching

Stretching improves flexibility, allowing you to move more easily. This will make it easier for you to reach down to tie your shoes or look over your shoulder when you back the car out of your driveway. You should do stretching activities after your muscles are warmed up — for example, after strength training. Stretching your muscles before they are warmed up may cause injury.

Tips to Help You get Moving

What are some tips to help me get moving?

Fit it into a busy schedule

- If you can't set aside one block of time, do short activities throughout the day, such as three 10-minute walks.

- Create opportunities for activity. Try parking your car farther away from where you are headed. If you ride the bus or train, get off one or two stops early and walk.

- Walk or bike to work or to the store.

- Use stairs instead of the elevator or escalator.

- Take breaks at work to stretch or take quick walks, or do something active with coworkers at lunch.

- Walk while you talk, if you're using a cellphone or cordless phone.

- Doing yard work or household chores counts as physical activity. Turn on some upbeat music to help you do chores faster and speed up your heart rate.

Make it fun

- Choose activities that you enjoy.

- Vary your activities, so you don't get bored. For instance, use different jogging, walking, or biking paths. Or bike one day, and jog the next.

- Reward yourself when you achieve your weekly goals. For instance, reward yourself by going to a movie.

- If you have children, make time to play with them outside. Set a good example!

- Plan active vacations that will keep you moving, such as taking tours and sightseeing on foot.

Make it social

- Join a hiking or running club.

- Go dancing with your partner or friends.

- Turn activities into social occasions — for example, go to a movie after you and a friend work out.

Overcome challenges

- Don't let cold weather keep you on the couch. You can find activities to do in the winter, such as indoor fitness classes or exercising to a workout video.

- If you live in a neighborhood where it is unsafe to be active outdoors, contact your local recreational center or church to see if they have indoor activity programs that you can join. You can also find ways to be active at home. For instance, you can do push-ups or lift hand weights. If you don't have hand weights, you can use canned foods or bottles filled with water or sand.

Don't expect to notice body changes right away. It can take weeks or months before you notice some of the changes from being physically active, such as weight loss. And keep in mind, many benefits of physical activity are happening inside you and you cannot see them.

Do I need to talk to my doctor before I start?

You should talk to your doctor before you begin any physical activity program if you:

- Have heart disease, had a stroke, or are at high risk for these diseases

- Have diabetes or are at high risk for diabetes

- Are obese (BMI of 30 or greater)

- Have an injury or disability

- Are pregnant

- Have a bleeding or detached retina, eye surgery, or laser treatment on your eye

- Have had recent hip surgery

How can I prevent injuries when I work out?

Being physically active is safe if you are careful. Take these steps to prevent injury:

- If you're not active at all or have a health problem, start your program with short sessions (5 to 10 minutes) of physical activity and build up to your goal. (Be sure to ask a doctor before you start if you have a health problem.)

- Use safety equipment such as a helmet for bike riding or supportive shoes for walking or jogging.

- Start every workout with a warm-up. If you plan to walk at a brisk pace, start by walking at an easy pace for 5 to 10 minutes. When you're done working out, do the same thing until your heart rate returns to normal.

- Drink plenty of fluids when you are physically active, even if you are not thirsty.

- Use sunscreen when you are outside.

- Always bend forward from the hips, not the waist. If you keep your back straight, you're probably bending the right way. If your back "humps," that's probably wrong.

- Stop your activity if you feel very out of breath, dizzy, nauseous, or have pain. If you feel tightness or pain in your chest or you feel faint or have trouble breathing, stop the activity right away and talk to your doctor.

Exercise should not hurt or make you feel really tired. You might feel some soreness, a little discomfort, or a bit weary. But you should not feel pain. In fact, in many ways, being active will probably make you feel better.

Can I stay active if I have a disability?

A disability may make it harder to stay active, but it shouldn't stop you. In most cases, people with disabilities can improve their flexibility, mobility, and coordination by becoming physically active. Getting regular physical activity can also help you stay independent by preventing illnesses, such as heart disease, that can make caring for yourself more difficult.

Even though you have a disability, you should still aim to meet the physical activity goals listed in how much physical activity should I do? Work with a doctor to develop a physical activity plan that works for you.

Reap the benefits of physical activities...

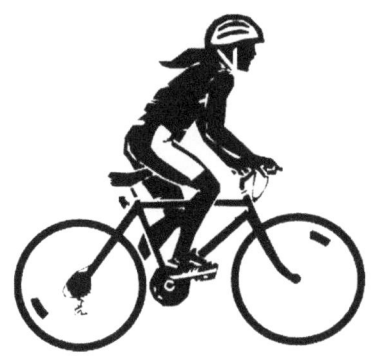

www.ingramcontent.com/pod-product-compliance
Lightning Source LLC
Chambersburg PA
CBHW050803290526
45792CB00008B/2309

*9 7 8 1 4 9 4 7 2 0 5 8 2 *